Stop the Stuttering!

Stop procrastinating and live life NOW!

DIET | EXERCISE

DON MIGUEL B.S. AND M.F.C.

DEDICATION

Stop the Stuttering is dedicated to all those who have made a significant impact on my life both mentally and physically.

To my mom, for all her heroism and strength and for being a source of great support and encouragement in all my efforts. To my sister, Laura, may you always live in our hearts, smiles and laughter – rest in peace. To my nieces, Jamilia and Jenelle, first born and first loved.

Finally, to Coach Cyrus Jones. Thank you for being there through thick and thin.

CONTENTS

1	Plan	1
2	Faith	9
3	80/20 Rules	13
4	Visualization	23
5	Decision	29
6	Path of Least Resistance	41
7	Repetition	51
	Final Thoughts	59
	About the Author	61

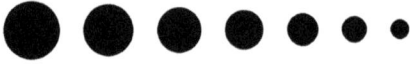

Plans are
nothing.
Planning is
everything.

Dwight D. Eisenhower

PLANNING

Successful people plan intentionally. Planning prepares you for success. Think back to the times in your life when you were successful at work, when you lost those first few pounds, when you met your weight loss goal or any other accomplishment. Did it involve a plan?

The Oxford English Dictionary defines plan as: An organized (and usually detailed) proposal according to which something is to be done; a scheme of action; a strategy; a schedule.

Plans can be ignored, but when used properly they can predict what the future should look like. Planning consists of positive reinforcement through concepts such as the 80/20 RULE, VISUALIZATION, DECISION, PATH OF LEAST RESISTANCE, FAITH, REPETITION. All of these will be discussed in the following pages to help with your plan.

Think of your diet and exercise as an expedition. You will need a map, the right amount of food, clothing, water, an expert guide and all the necessary tools to complete your journey. Just like an expedition, all of these things are needed to make a complete workout and dietary plan for weight loss.

If you don't plan,
plan to fail!

Taking 15-20 minutes every day for planning is critical for attaining your weight goals and the freedom you desire. Failure and disappointment often happen when you do not plan for success. You are the master of your destiny – don't give up that control. By taking control and responsibility for your actions, you will create your weight loss success. A favorite quote by which I live is, "A body in motion stays in motion."

Creating a practical plan is critical. Here are some points to consider when making your plan:

1. Write out your plan. This makes it more concrete and attainable.
2. Guide your plan with "SMART" – Specific, Measurable, Achievable, Realistic and Time-bound.
3. Plan 30-60 days ahead to allow for trial and error.
4. Group yourself with positive, agreeable people who have a similar goal and who are willing to keep you accountable.
5. Commit to meeting at least three times a week with your group.
6. Positively visualize doing and accomplishing your plan daily.

A body in motion
stays in motion.

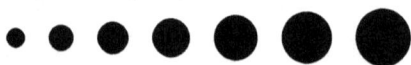

7. Be candid with yourself about your struggles and successes.

8. Believe you can accomplish your plans and have faith in your positive visualization.

9. Self-praise, and celebrate every accomplishment from small to big, but within reason.

10. Repeat until you get it right! There is nothing wrong with repetition.

Without a written practical plan, your goals are just thoughts. Thoughts are subject to change with shifting emotions and daily life. Too many well intended thoughts sit on the shelves of our brains collecting dust. Let your motivation inspire true action, make a determined plan! Don't linger in analysis paralysis, just start!

Still not convinced? The man who says he can and the man who says he cannot are both right. Be the man or woman who says, "I can!" This book is not meant to facilitate limitations but to inspire faith and hope in those looking for it.

Be your best before and after success story of weight loss. In my experience, clients who lose weight gain freedom. Freedom from poor health, lack of self-confidence, fear, doubt, insecurities, negative criticism and sleeplessness. Successful weight loss makes you more attractive and interesting. Compliments will flow to you and the wind will be at your back. No obstacle will be too big to conquer when you have met your weight loss goals. Others will want what you have, and they will want to know how you did it.

People are always looking to relate. You can be a positive influence in their lives. You can capture the aura of success!

If you are not building the body you want, then you are tearing it down.

So take leadership of yourself and use my sample schedule plan to create your own:

"In three months time, I want the ability to walk 3 miles in 30 minutes, or run a 5K in one hour."

The idea is to measure your performance or improvement against your last efforts. Use your first walk as a benchmark and decrease the time it takes to complete the activity but do so realistically. Just as babies learn to walk in small steps, most people progress in the same way. You do not have to be an athlete to become successful.

List 5 eating habits you would like to change today:

1)_____

2)_____

3)_____

4)_____

5)_____

List 5 exercise plans you would like to begin today:

1)_____

2)_____

3)_____

4)_____

5)_____

My dream is
my reality
my reality is
my dream.

Donald Trump

FAITH

I define faith as: taking the time to understand someone else's perspective who has experienced dieting and exercise success and learning how it can be applied into your life.

Faith is like many intangible concepts such as patience, love, forgiveness. Faith has no limits; you can have faith without measure. Faith is to success what choice is to decision. Faith gives us hope that our desires can be accomplished. With faith you do not need proof, just hope and belief. The Scripture says, "It is impossible to please God without faith." Faith is the "confident assurance that what we hope for is going to happen. It is the evidence of things we cannot yet see."

The truth is that our desires cannot manifest themselves without the application of faith. Desires and success cannot be accomplished without faith.

Planning and faith seem all well and good, but how do you get started with your plan? The expression *"the hardest thing is getting started"* has truth in weight loss, but I say the hardest thing is believing in yourself. You must believe that you can accomplish your goals of eating right, working out consistently, achieving weight loss and keeping the weight off. My "7 Steps to success and freedom through diet and exercise" will help you with this process.

What's one of the secrets to success through my plan? Success is 80% mental and 20% physical. My 7 well-laid steps encourage each successive step simply by you doing. By making a DECISION that you can and the CHOICE that you will, you exercise your faith that makes up part of the 80% of weight loss success.

Unfortunately, the 80% does not make the 20% physical simply disappear. The 20% is needed to make your dream a reality. After all, "Faith without work is dead." Now, let's get started, a body in motion stays in motion!

7 exercise steps to develop your faith:

Dream

Desire

Imagine/Visualize

Believe

Decide

Persist

Practice gratitude or be thankful

How have you exercised your faith today?
List 5 ways:

1)_____

2)_____

3)_____

4)_____

5)_____

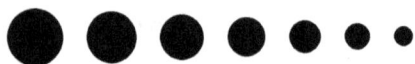

Insanity is
doing the
same thing
over and over
again and
expecting
different results.

Albert Einstein

80/20 RULES

Successful people make "the rules of life" play to their strengths and advantages.

Interestingly enough, many diet and exercise books put the 20% physical above the 80% mental. Without a strong emphasis on the mental side of weight-loss, your journey will be confusing and your goals unattainable.

To do something physical over and over again without results would be insane. By making your weight-loss plan 80% mental and 20% physical, you ensure that you are maximizing your potential and not wasting your time.

Concentrating 80% effort on the mental side of weight loss has contributed to many a success story. It has set many free from the failures and frustrations of unattained desires.

The 80/20 Rule really is important for planning your own successful weight loss story. The Rule gives structure to your plan by prioritizing the right state of mind. We all must win in our minds before we can direct our minds at winning in the world.

In my early thirties, I was a finely tuned track and field athlete. During that time, I truly discovered how important a positive mindset and attitude was in realizing my true potential. Successful performances became more mental than physical – 80/20 to be exact!

You have to have the ability to make decisions and choices, not have them made for you, in order to become successful. If you overly concentrate on the physical, your mental state will not be strong enough to enforce the application of your goals and plan.

Successful weight loss begins and ends, is won or lost, in the mind. To ensure your success, refer to the practical plan steps in PLANNING numbers one through ten, for guidance and repeat Steps two through seven. VISUALIZATION, DECISION, PATH OF LEAST RESISTANCE, REPETITION. Repetition strengthens the image of something in your mind.

Remember, you fail only when you give up and stop trying.

Nutrition is the interaction of food within the body and follows the 80/20 RULES for weight loss success. It includes ingestion, digestion, absorption, transport, metabolism and exercise. Without adequate planning, the 80%, nutrition will not work well enough for you.

Physical weight loss is the process of breaking down the body and relying on three basic food groups – protein, carbohydrates and fats – to put back what was lost (see the food pyramid chart below). Without appropriate food from the three basic groups, you will not have the energy to sustain workouts, the necessary nutrients to fuel muscle growth or your desired weight loss.

Consult a nutrition expert or certified nutritionist for a comprehensive and specific eating plan. The nutritionist will help you navigate misleading information from fad diets and unqualified individuals. They can also help you work through food allergies or structure your diet along personal choices (vegetarian or religious).

Another great place to get started is www.mypyramid.gov.

Keep it simple, otherwise, it's not worth your time. My basic practical steps are:

- Eat fruits, vegetables and lean meats.
- Stay away from processed foods.
- If you dine out, eat a small snack prior to leaving home or drink lots of water before eating. Maybe even ask to have your

meal without the trimmings or split it with someone.

- Plan and decide your approach before you get to dinner.

Successful weight loss is a journey rather than a destination. If you truly desire successful weight loss, you will do what it takes!

My 7 tips for successful weight loss are:

1. Believe you can do it.
2. See yourself losing the weight.
3. Do it for yourself.
4. Be patient with the process.
5. Accept your failures, but do not adopt them.
6. Be positive and reward positive behavior within reason.
7. Exercise or be active.

Ideal 80/20 Rule

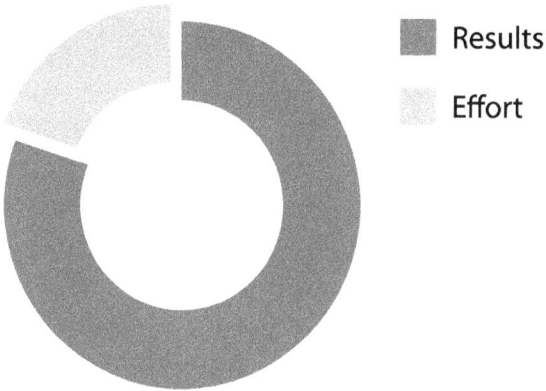

The above chart shows that 80% of your results come from 20% of your efforts. IDEAL.

While below shows 20% of your results come from 80% of your efforts. NOT IDEAL.

Not Ideal 80/20 Rule

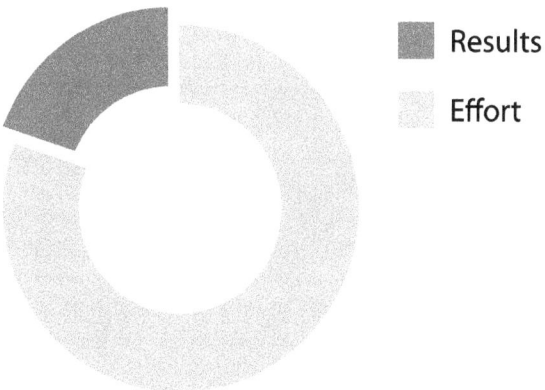

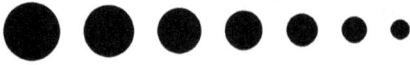

80 percent
of your results
should come from 20
percent
of your activities.

Daily eating suggestion consists of 5-6 small meals that are consumed every 2 hours:

Breakfast

Snack

Lunch

Snack

Dinner

Snack

Additional information can be found at www.mypyramid.gov.

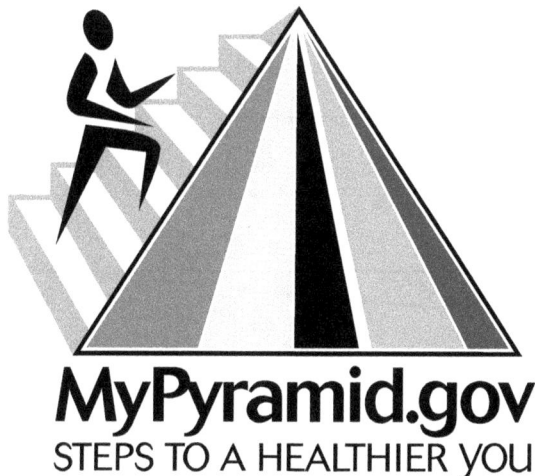

MyPyramid.gov
STEPS TO A HEALTHIER YOU

List 5 eating habits you would like to change today:

1)_____

2)_____

3)_____

4)_____

5)_____

List 5 reasons you want to change the habits:

1)_____

2)_____

3)_____

4)_____

5)_____

Successful weight loss means taking responsibility for your actions – both eating and how you exercise. Do you eat more than you exercise? Do you exercise at high or low intensity?

Focus on what's working and where you have seen improvements: move up from 8 pushups per session to 17; run one lap without stopping; show up for workouts on-time and prepared.

Remain positive every step of the journey and remember that big accomplishments start small.

If you reward yourself for positive action, you will get more positive results. If you punish yourself for negative action, you get more negative results. We condition ourselves based upon positive and negative reinforcement, so, reinforce the positive!

Visualization is
integral to
imagination
and supported
by Faith.

Don Miguel

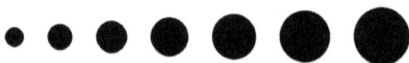

VISUALIZATION

Visualization is like a small, and skinny kid with big feet. Although the kid starts off awkward, he eventually grows to 6'5" and into a proportionate body. Apply this simile to visualizing your success. Your goals and application of your plan may seem awkward at first; but, as you grow and develop, they become a natural experience from intentional behavior.

When I decided to write Stop the Stuttering, I visualized that I would finish what I started. Then I made a plan and followed it through, even though writing felt awkward at first. True to my personality, I finish what I start and so can you.

To start my book, I needed a table of contents to complete the initial visualization in my mind. As I wrote each section, I could look upon my table of contents for visual conformation that I was completing my goal. The visual conformation fed my desire to be successful.

It was important for me to mentally see and physically feel all seven steps in order to complete my writing. So I visualized a skeletal frame that required muscles and tendons. My visualization helped expand and fuel my desire daily. You will experience a similar and successful result when you visualize yourself completing my 7 Steps.

I visualized my entire book from start to finish, starting with my plan to write out all 7 Steps and post them on my desktop. I believed that it could and would be done no matter what.

After two years of due diligence, practicing the 80/20 rule and visualizing, my efforts were realized. I decided not to give up or take the path of least resistance. Writing did not come naturally to me, but I filled myself with determination not to give up simply because my desires had obstacles in the pathway.

You cannot improve your visualization immediately, working to make it happen requires faith. Hope and belief will help you realize your visualization. Just as you need faith to visualize, visualization will increase your faith. Meditate and think over your visualizations. Let yourself feel success. Practicing visualization will give you focus, clarity and increased ability to implement the 80% mental part of your plan.

Do not avoid visualizing your success! Seeing yourself completing the plan is not cheating; it will help your outlook as you undergo my 7 Steps plan!

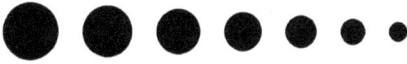

Limitation lives in the
mind and with words,
shape your desire.

Don Miguel

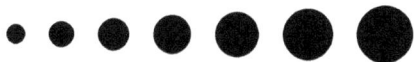

As faith in your visualization increases, your self-image will change. You will feel up to the task of weight loss and will do away with negative energy. Use visualization wisely to construct the reality you want, then follow the positive steps you have visualized.

7 practical steps to better visualization:

Get the pictures
Repetition
Faith
Focus
Consistency
Patience
Practice
Plan
Silence/Meditation

Avoid unproductive and destructive applications of visualization like:

Day dreaming
Harming yourself and others
Thinking in negative, instead of positive, terms
Reliving past negative experiences
Fears about the future

What are 5 things must you visualize to be successful at attaining your weight loss goal?

1)_____

2)_____

3)_____

4)_____

5)_____

Struggles of life
are the
greatest equalizer.

Don Miguel

DECISION

Decision is the beginning of all great victories. I learned from a young age that I am responsible for my decisions, both good and bad. Also I learned that talk is limited. Telling others about something does not make it happen.

At age eleven, I failed my high school entrance exam. My parents reinforced that, if I did not pass it the second time, I would be a street worker for the rest of my life. Although their reinforcement seemed cruel, my parents understood what motivated me. They used the situation to increase my desire to work harder and succeed. My older brother and sister had passed the exam on their first attempt, so the pressure was on me to perform.

I can recall visualizing unwanted images of being a street worker. It was not the path that I wanted to live or how I had pictured my future. I had to make a decision to change the course of my life; I had to decide to pass that entrance exam. So I committed myself to studying hard and took advantage of the prep classes offered. I was determined not to be a street worker.

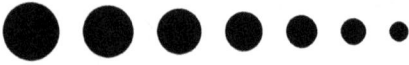

Nothing is written unless you write it.

Lawrence of Arabia

Through determination and patience, I succeeded in passing my exam. The experience helped shape my will. I decided not to give up until my visualizations and plans came into reality. Come what may, I would not deviate from my plan; I would not let my emotions and others get me off-course.

As a fitness expert, I made the decision years ago that I would never have a belly as long I lived. I remain committed to doing what it takes and finding ways to make a fit life my reality. I made a decision and continue to make it daily. I persevere through adversity and do not make excuses.

People who have made a decision about attaining their weight loss goals do not take the path of least resistance. When its raining and cold outside, they exercise inside. When you make good decisions, you can be who you want and go where you want.

Exercising your will by deciding to eat right and exercise, even when you don't feel like it, has an empowering effect on both mental and physical aspects of your life. Remember, "success begets success."

Don't be afraid to fail!

Decisions cause success and freedom; whereas, Indecision causes failures and frustrations.

The following chart visualizes how making a decision helps guide you in the direction of success whereas not making a decision pushes you in the direction of failure.

Decision vs. Indecision

DECISION	INDECISION
Faith	Fear
Knowledge	Confusion
Commitment	Doubt
Patience	Little to no control
Positive	Ill-Health
Control	Defensiveness
Proactive	Procrastination
Offense	Mediocrity
Peace	Hopelessness
Hope	Regret
Choice	Shame
Plan	Pride
Power	Passivity
Action	Worry
Courage	Failure
Prioritize	Condemnation
Persistence	Frustration
Determination	
Freedom	
Self Discipline	
Enthusiasm	
Dedication	

Successful behavior builds on itself, as does negative behavior. Each gives back as much as you put in. So invest in positive decisions and move towards success!

Three life-changing phrases to adopt:

I can
I will
I am

Create a pledge of, *"I can, I will, I am"* and repeat it twice daily – when you first get up and before you go to sleep. Follow my example below.

Daily pledge to repeat when you feel like giving up:

I am strong. I am healthy. I am Fit.

I will make healthy food choices.
I will be active.

I will be hard-working, patient, and dedicated.

I will take responsibility for my actions.
I will respect and believe in myself.

I am strong. I am healthy. I am Fit.

List your top 5 exercise and eating decisions:

1)_____

2)_____

3)_____

4)_____

5)_____

List your positive eating and fitness promises:

1)_____

2)_____

3)_____

4)_____

5)_____

Make a decision NOW to continue your weight loss success journey!

Signs of people that have chosen to be successful at weight loss:

1. Eat breakfast
2. Make no excuses
3. Have a vision
4. Do not fear the unknown
5. Do not stay in their "comfort zone"
6. Refuse to follow diet fads
7. Don't skip meals
8. Keep an eating journal
9. Believe in themselves
10. Set attainable goals
11. Notice and celebrate the small successes
12. Don't argue for their limitation
13. Not critical of themselves or others
14. Don't give up easily or at the first failure
15. Open-mined
16. Understand the difference between weight loss and how to keep it off

Fear is an enemy acting on your decisions! Fear of failure will inhibit you from attaining your success and freedom. One of the best warnings I received after I finished my college track career was that fear smothers talent and ability.

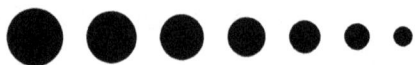

I decide
to see the world
for how
I want it to be.

Don Miguel

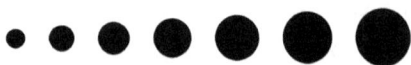

Many people fail because they are afraid of what others may think of their failure. In reality, failure is essential to everyone's success. It may be the failure of someone else or that of your own.

Failure is not always bad. Determined and successful people learn from failure and become stronger because of it. Three famous examples are Babe Ruth, Thomas Edison and Abraham Lincoln. All three men failed numerous times but understood failure was temporary.

My personal experience with failure is not different from that of most people, but what separates me from many is willpower. I refuse to let my decisions be thwarted by circumstances or obstacles. They only help me develop strength, character and perseverance.

I believe that successful weight loss is important to you. Whatever is making you unhappy is temporary, you can decide to change it. Don't settle for less than the completion of your goals. You don't have to give in and you are not defeated. Your past or present situation should not determine how you see yourself or your future.

I have four words to help your willpower and decision making abilities:

COURAGE – to do the right thing when you are alone, to change, to be a leader, to make a decision and choose to fulfill your potential. You must be like a leader, courageous and full of conviction. Be one who dares to believe differently and against the odds until your visions and passions have been attained.

ENTHUSIASM – to be excited by the thought of successfully completing all 7 Steps, and undiscouraged about any failures or obstacles that are ahead. They mean you are headed in a forward direction, toward losing the weight, eating better and just being excited about NOW. Every moment is yours to seize and conquer. Don't wait until you lose the weight to get excited. Be excited every step of the way. Think of it as the long awaited vacation. Every moment and everyday leading up to your success should be full of energy and excitement. Get excited, you are changing the way you look and feel. Enthusiasm is contagious; it will inspire those around you.

COMMITMENT – to the body and lifestyle you desire, to living life above average and to avoid mediocrity. Lead by example. Everyone loves to hear about an underdog succeeding

- the kid with one arm who rides his bike 100 miles or the person who weighed 500 pounds dropping down to 150. What is stopping you from creating your story? The world is ready for it. Commit to your plan and make strong decisions!

DEDICATION – to yourself, to family and to being responsible. Dedicate yourself to following my 7 Steps, losing the weight and keeping it off! I challenge you to dedicate yourself to your plan and to attaining your goals!

The defining point in every situation is a decision. Every person who successfully loses weight must make strong decisions every day. Keep courage, enthusiasm, commitment and dedication in your mind. Do not be afraid of failure. The only way to make your goals happen is to begin.

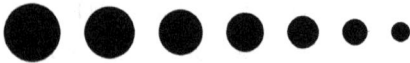

He that can't
endure the bad
will not live
to see
the good.

Yiddish Proverb

PATH OF LEAST RESISTANCE

As you read this section, I will help you identify what to avoid, as well as, what to do when you feel uninspired or unfocused. I will advise you on what to look for when selecting a trainer or fitness expert, what language to expect when getting started, what places to visit to keep your experience interesting and how to stay in the game and win.

A wise man once said, "Desire is the starting point of all achievement, and if what you have is truly a desire, you will get yourself compelled to do something about it."

Success begins with desire and a flexible plan as we work my 7 Steps to weight loss. Many media sources and publications try to get you to take a path of least resistance in your diet and exercise regime. They do not ask you to think about what you are doing, just to do something that seems easy enough. By following paths of least resistance, we fail without really trying.

Don't give up! Giving up proves that everyone was right about you and that you are not able to finish what you start. I think and believe differently. That's why you are on Step 6 of my book. You have made it this far because you

The tendency of the masses is towards mediocrity.

Aldous Huxley

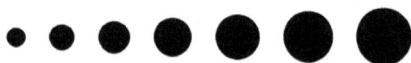

believed in yourself and so do I. Do not justify bad behaviors or fall into cycles of negative reinforcement.

If you are inactive, make consequences for yourself. Get your friends involved, have them withhold something you value if you do not meet your goals. Expose all the escape routes you have made for yourself and shut them off. I know of many people who started on their journey only to go back to their negative habits. When things get tough, repeat my pledge. You can attain success and freedom.

People such as yourself, who avoid the path of least resistance are committed to continuous personal growth and development.

Dedicated people go the extra mile, finish what they start and seek to improve upon their best. They are qualified because of their desires, see the big picture, give without expecting to receive, live passionately, never give up and have faith as their confidant.

Signs of people that are not successful at weight loss:

1.   Don't eat breakfast
2.   Make excuses
3.   Lacks vision

4. Fearful of the unknown
5. Ruled by their comfort level
6. Follow diet fads
7. Skip meals
8. Don't keep an eating journal
9. Doubt themselves
10. Set goals too high
11. Don't notice the small successes
12. Argue for their limitation- I can't, I hate, I will try...
13. Critical of themselves and others
14. Give up easily or at the first failure
15. Not open-mined
16. Don't understand the difference between weight loss and how to keep it off

Repeat your pledge daily if you feel like giving up:

I am strong. I am healthy. I am Fit.
I will make healthy food choices.
I will be active.
I will be hard-working, patient, and dedicated.
I will take responsibility for my actions.
I will respect and believe in myself.
I am strong. I am healthy. I am Fit.

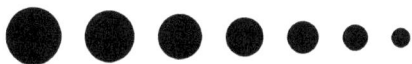

Pursuit is the proof of desire.

Mike Murdock

The defining point in every situation is a decision.

Don Miguel

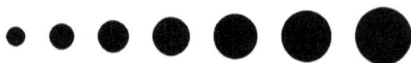

Before beginning any exercise program, I recommend you consult with your doctor. Then consult with a qualified fitness professional. The following list provides tips on how to chose a qualified fitness professional.

1. Observe, then observe some more.
2. Ask someone who has had a successful experience with a trainer.
3. Is the trainer result driven?
4. Does the trainer practice safety?
5. Does the trainer take the time to explain and answer your questions with consideration to your concerns?
6. Is the trainer dedicated, passionate and current?
7. Don't base your decision on the fitness of the trainer, but the fitness of his/her clients.
8. Make a well-informed decision and not a fear based one.

The following is a list of things you will commonly experience in a workout session. Each is important because it is where you begin to understand the general idea of weight or resistance training and how to establish benchmarks.

Sets

Reps

Rest

Body fat ratio

Resting Heart Rate

Interval training

Probability

Progressive

Variety

Basic, intermediate and advance fitness levels

Three weeks then change workouts

Group or individual motivation

Best exercises: push-ups (modified-regular), walking lunges, planks, jumping jacks, pull-ups (modified-regular)

Body resistance, plyometrics, weights,

Other modalities: medicine ball, kettle bell, jump ropes, bands, tubing, dumb bells, body bar, BOSU, gliders,

For variety here are a few suggestions to consider:

Crossfit
Karate
Velocity
Mixed Martial Arts

Boxing gyms
Dance and exercise studios

Adults are encouraged to have minimum of 30 minutes of moderate to intense activity 4-6 days a week.

Take notes on your workouts; write down all your exercises. Taking notes generates a great visual aide of accomplishment. It can keep you motivated and confident.

Write down exercises from your favorite workout and exercise DVDs. They are a great place to start. In your own words, notate all exercises, so when the time comes to review, it's easy to remember what to do.

Investigate what motivates other people to be successful at weight loss. Even try applying their methods in good faith. Take the time and effort to try out a different fitness class or professional trainers so you can discover what motivates others and how they enjoy working out.

Practice is
repetition,
performance
made perfect.

Don Miguel

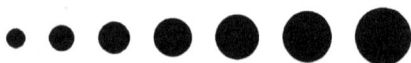

REPETITION

Take a moment, close your eyes and imagine yourself on stage or in a meeting with total strangers. You are expected to comment on a subject you know little to nothing about, but are required to comment anyway. I regularly experienced this while growing up. Unfortunately, I had a problem speaking publicly because I stuttered.

Repetition is to stuttering what my 7 Steps are to success and freedom through diet and exercise. Repetition also creates enthusiasm. It prepares the 80% mind for the 20% action.

I was called names and teased constantly. I believe God gave me ways of adjusting to the challenges He knew I would have to face. It was a test to see if I would succumb or rise to the occasion or confrontation. I rose up, but not without some amount of trepidation and, sometimes, failure. In the beginning, I solved everything with my fist or whatever I could get my hand on, because I was overly frustrated. As I got older, I learned how to use my stuttering to my advantage, because people would take pity on me and either stop and listen or try to help me finish what I had to say.

Don't be afraid to fail!

In completing this book, I can say that stuttering and never giving up have made me a better and more effective communicator. Stuttering has made me more understanding and willing to help others. It taught me that repetition is not a bad thing, but something that helps with better understanding the world around me. I embraced my stuttering and decided that it was more of an asset than a hindrance. I embrace repetition daily and call it my own. If I did that, then so can you.

I can imagine that the challenge of weight loss is fearful for a lot of people. You're tackling an issue that is both confusing and personal, and you can't seem to get it right no matter how many times or how hard you try. If losing weight was easy, we would all be fit and slim.

Having a sport and fitness background, I understand fitness success and failure. When you fall, get back up and keep going. Learning from your past mistakes and repeating the good decisions will lead to success.

To be good at sports or the arts, one must practice. Practice is repetition, performance made perfect. It's repeating the pledge daily, and rehearsing your visualization. It is not taking the path of least resistance but repeating steps 1-7 of my book. Through repetition we can

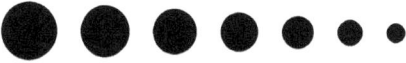

Desire is possibility seeking expression.

Ralph Waldo Emerson

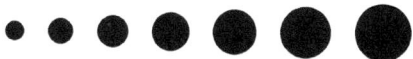

create positive habits that will, with enough repetition, become second nature to us.

REPETITION is a wash cycle. You have a number of different options, but one result.

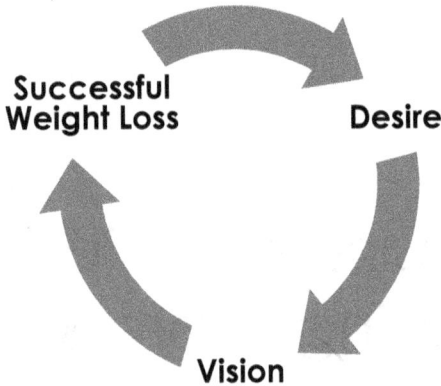

Successful Weight Loss — **Desire** — **Vision** (cycle diagram)

Birth Desire – Possible Vision – Consistency and Dedication = Successful Weight Loss

Separate yourself from the discouraging crowd and take the road less traveled. Go the extra mile. Form a supportive team, but please no one but yourself, because its your one and only life.

It's also your plan; your faith exercised. It's you who must play by the rules. It's your vision; your decision; your path repeated that will produce your desire for freedom and success through diet and exercise.

My great concern is not whether you have failed, but whether you are content with your failure.

Abraham Lincoln

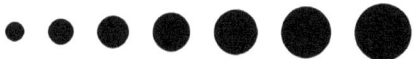

Let's start from the top... what have you learned, how must you start and what must you do?

Plan - first plan.

Faith - exercise your belief.

80/20 Rules - know the rules or play by the rules. of engagement. Play to win.

Visualization - keep it basic or stick to the fundamentals.

Decision - make active and intentional decisions.

Path of Least Resistance – self-discipline.

Repetition – make and learn from mistakes. Then repeat steps 1-7.

Daily pledge to repeat when you feel like giving up:

I am strong. I am healthy. I am Fit.

I will make healthy food choices.
I will be active.

I will be hard-working, patient, and dedicated.

I will take responsibility for my actions.
I will respect and believe in myself.

I am strong. I am healthy. I am Fit.

RISE AND RISE AGAIN
UNTIL
LAMBS BECOME LIONS.

Robin Hood the Movie, 2010

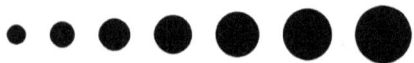

FINAL THOUGHTS

I am finally able to realize my dream of completing my first book. For me, writing has never been my strong suit. I can remember my breakthrough came five years ago when I was encouraged to "just" put all my thoughts down on paper without concern for grammar or punctuation. This was the first step in building my confidence to write and freely express myself. The rest as they say "is history!" I had faith in myself and that of others, which gave me additional inspiration to write.

The rest was easy because of my passion for fitness and helping people succeed.

If you have enjoyed this book,
or if it has had an impact on your life,
I would like to hear from you.

For more information about
Don Miguel's book, consulting,
and coaching: Individual & Corporate
Please contact me at:

MediaFit Communications
25 Highland Park Village Suite 100-726
Dallas, TX 75205

Or visit my web site:
www.StopTheStutteringBook.com

ABOUT THE AUTHOR

Don Miguel serves as the CEO and Chairman of the Board of Fit-for-Me Foundation. He guides the organization's educational efforts to advocate and advance programs and services directed at bettering the lives of young people. The programs focus on fitness, wellness and addressing the ever-increasing obesity problem in America. Don Miguel represents Fit-for-Me Foundation at public policy, fitness and wellness industry, and health-related industry events. He also frequently speaks with members of the media and other organizations about Fit-for-Me Foundation's efforts.

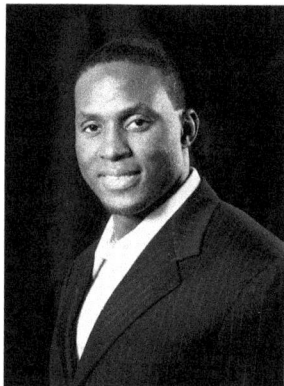

Don Miguel has more than sixteen years experience in fitness and wellness. He was named one of the Top 20 Trainers for Town Sports International, parent company of Washington Sports Club / New York Sports Club / Boston Sports Club / Philadelphia Sports Club, and Best Trainer in the tri-state area of Virginia, Maryland and Washington, D.C.

Don Miguel has a passion for changing the lives of people through physical fitness and wellness, which is evident in his foundation's mission, purpose and goals.

He is a certified to promote healthy behaviors in children through his membership in the Cooper Aerobics Institute. He is also affiliated IDEA, where he is an IDEA Master Level Personal Fitness Trainer.

Don Miguel holds a B.S. degree in Health Science from Lincoln University. His dedication to fitness is reflected through his fitness and wellness endeavors and on-going educational pursuits. In fitness and wellness, Don Miguel thinks of everyone as winners. He embraces a commitment to an active lifestyle and has fun doing it.

NOTES

NOTES

NOTES

NOTES

NOTES

NOTES

NOTES

NOTES

www.ingramcontent.com/pod-product-compliance
Lightning Source LLC
Chambersburg PA
CBHW052105270326
41931CB00012B/2890